Reply to Warnock

by

Richard Higginson

Ethics Tutor at St. John's College, Durham

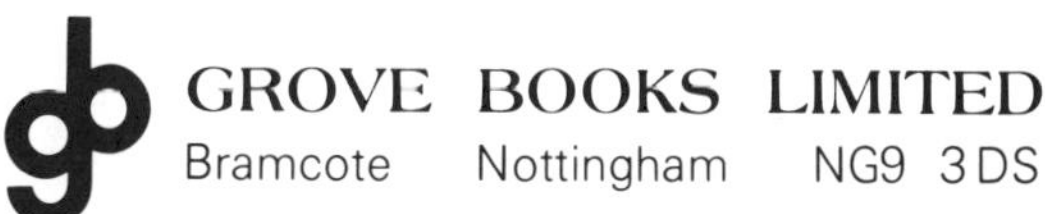
GROVE BOOKS LIMITED
Bramcote Nottingham NG9 3DS

CONTENTS

ACKNOWLEDGEMENTS

I would like to thank the many groups with whom I have dicussed the issues contained in the Warnock Report, in particular student groups at Cranmer Hall. They have been an aid and stimulus to my thinking. Thanks also to my colleague Michael Vasey for the loan of his word-processor in the preparation of the draft for this booklet.

THE COVER PICTURE

. . . is devised by Greg Foster

First Impression October 1986

ISSN 0305–4241

ISBN 1 85174 037 6

1. WARNOCK: A WELL-WORN BATTLEGROUND?

It is with a certain amount of reluctance that I have become persuaded that it is right to take up the pen and write a Grove Booklet on the issues raised by the Warnock Report.

The first inhibiting factor is that I am aware that a great deal has already been written upon this subject. The last two years have seen a veritable wealth of publications, major and minor, Christian and secular, following in the wake of the Warnock Report. Before the Report came out several Grove Booklets discussing issues which came to the fore with Warnock had already appeared.[1] I have myself made a previous venture into this area of debate.[2] Readers may share this strong sense of *dejà vu* on being confronted with another exploration of the issues of artificial fertilization and embryology.

The second reason for my reluctance is that involvement in discussion on the Warnock issues has been a far from happy experience. The tone of debate has been sharp, if not fiercely polemical. Not only in the public and Parliamentary arena, but also in Christian—even evangelical—circles, bitter words have been spoken, wounding allegations made and received. There has sometimes appeared to be a heartless lack of compassion for childless couples on the one side, or a chilling lack of respect for the embryo on the other. And too much of the response to the Warnock Report has partaken of an unduly simple 'for or against' mentality.

Why then have I overcome these feelings of reluctance in order to add to the volume of words on Warnock? For a variety of reason. Partly because the issues remain very much alive: the Warnock Report is still on the table, the present Government seems decidedly reluctant to legislate upon it, and so the future of various practices described in it remains uncertain, though, with each passing month of legislative inactivity, these techniques become a little more securely established and the clock that much more difficult to turn back. Partly because I feel I may be able to offer a contribution which, while strongly committed and sharply critical of certain practices, seeks to enter sympathetically into the very real dilemmas entailed in these issues, and to some extent to depolemicize the debate. Partly because the Warnock Report is a substantial document on moral issues of major topical significance and it would seem to be a culpable omission if the Grove Ethics series failed to make a response to these issues as a whole. And partly because mingled with my feelings of reluctance is a certain abiding fascination . . .

[1] Notably Oliver O'Donovan, *The Christian and the Unborn Child* (Grove Ethics Booklet no. 1); D. Gareth Jones, *Genetic Engineering* (no. 25); and David Ison, *Artificial Insemination by Donor* (no. 52).

[2] Richard Higginson, 'What's Wrong with Warnock', *Anvil,* 2:1 (1985) pp.9-23.

2. CHILDLESS COUPLES AND ROOTLESS CHILDREN

Most of the practices on which the Warnock Report comments pre-dated its work by some years. Artificial Insemination by Donor has been practised in this country since the Second World War and has been quite widely, if unevenly, available since 1960. The birth of the first 'test-tube' baby, Louise Brown, in 1978 followed nearly a decade of research into *in vitro* fertilization. Public attention on the field of artificial insemination and embryology seems to have increased considerably after that dramatic event. In fact the IVF pioneers, Robert Edwards and Patrick Steptoe, had been requesting legislative guidelines in an unclear situation for many years; but it was not until July 1982 that a Committee of Inquiry under Lady Mary Warnock was set up

> 'To consider recent and potential developments in medicine and science related to human fertilization and embryology; to consider what policies and safeguards should be applied, including consideration of the social, ethical and legal implications of these developments; and to make recommendations.'[1]

The Committee worked quickly, and published its Report in June 1984. Chapters 3 to 8 of the Report are headed 'Techniques for the Alleviation of Infertility'. It is a curious use of the word *alleviation.* One would have thought that a more accurate description of these techniques is the overcoming of childlessness or the circumvention of infertility. This is not just a semantic point, because it draws attention to a striking omission in the Report. The Report cites the familiar estimate that about one couple in ten are thought to suffer from infertility. It outlines the scope of the problem, while lamenting the lack of accurate statistics on the subject. But there is no exploration of the various reasons why some couples are unable to conceive children, other than mention of the purely physical factors which can lead in the direction of one artificial technique rather than another. Yet it would surely have been relevant to point out that psychological factors can affect performance of the act of sexual intercourse, the emission of semen and therefore the chances of conception; that damage to a woman's fallopian tubes is often caused through the effects of a previous abortion, use of the coil as a contraceptive device, or sexually transmitted diseases; and that sometimes there is no discernible reason why a couple cannot conceive (fertilization being something of a random affair, certain couples are persistently unlucky). The intention of drawing attention to these factors would not be to heap scorn, blame or pity on the individuals concerned. Rather, attempting to identify the causes of infertility in particular cases should be the prelude to finding an appropriate therapy; and for some couples resort to sexual therapy, repair of the fallopian tubes or simply a willingness to go on trying would appear to be the appropriate step before artificial techniques for overcoming childlessness are seriously considered. Doubtless most couples do go through such preliminary stages first. What is strange is that the Report rushes on to the artificial techniques so quickly.

[1] *Report of the Committee of Inquiry into Human Fertilisation and Embryology* (henceforth *'Warnock Report'*) (HMSO, 1984) para. 1.2.

The fact remains that a substantial minority of couples, many of whom are in no sense to blame for their infertility problem, even after resort to therapy of an appropriate kind, still find themselves saddled with the sad reality of childlessness. (There are of course some couples who choose not to have children, but one assumes them to be a minority within the category of childless couples). There is no doubting that involuntary childlessness causes suffering. Part of the pressure to have children is a social pressure: it is something that most couples do, the joys and satisfactions which it brings usually seem to outweigh the strains and sorrows, and couples who do not have children clearly fall outside the social norm. The excitement that news of an expected birth brings to the extended family, especially grandparents, is paralleled by the disappointment caused by a failure to conceive. But a greater part of the pressure to conceive probably comes from within: individually and as a couple, the desire to perpetuate one's line and to consummate one's sexual relationship through the creation of a child, whom one can nurture and cherish, is an extremely strong human instinct.

Hairs have been split over whether the desire to bear children constitutes a need or a want. For most couples it is a want which, if unsatisfied, creates a deep emotional need. It is not of course crucial to life; nor should it be crucial to the survival of a loving marital relaionship; but it leaves a huge hole amidst the realizations of the usual expectations of that relationship. Childlessness creates much misery, and if new techniques appear to hold out the hope of overcoming it, we are duty-bound to give them at the very least sympathetic consideration.

In the Bible, childnessness is viewed as a great human sorrow, and sometimes as a sign of divine disfavour.[1] But just as God takes away, so also he delights to give and to restore. The joy which Hannah experienced at the birth of Samuel will find echoes in many couples who have thought they were infertile and then pleasantly discovered otherwise! God's concern for the childless widow is shown in his provision of levirite marriage to ensure a progeny.[2] Even resort by Abraham and Jacob to *natural* insemination of their barren wives' slave-girls is not recorded as meeting with God's disapproval. A Christian doctor who is sympathetic to the Warnock recommendations has suggested to me that 'Rachel and Sarah would be leaning over the battlements cheering Lady Warnock on at the moment'!

Because of the suffering which childlessness brings, and because of the obvious immediate joy which circumvention of infertility through the use of new artificial techniques has undeniably brought, the case for pressing ahead with these techniques and making them available as widely as possible is seen by some as unanswerable. To raise questions about the moral propriety and psychological advisability of resorting to such techniques is to run the risk of being accused of legalistic nit-picking and lack of compassion for the childless couple. It is especially difficult if one is oneself able to conceive children through natural means and appears to be saying 'No' to a pleasure that one has oneself been privileged to enjoy. Yet the case for pressing ahead should not be assumed to be proven incontestably too quickly. It is not just moral prudes or kill-joys

[1] See, e.g., Gen. 20.17-18; 2 Sam. 6.23.

[2] See Deut. 25.5-6. Here the emphasis falls on the importance of having an *heir.*

who harbour doubts about these techniques; indeed, the scruples of some childless couples are such that they are not prepared to resort to them. In the words of the Warnock Report, the reason why the Committee was set up was because

> 'Society's views on the new techniques were divided between pride in the technological achievement, pleasure at the new-found means to relieve, at least for some, the unhappiness of infertility, and unease at the apparently uncontrollable advance of science, bringing with it new possibilities for manipulating the early stages of human development.'[1]

In short, there was anxiety about the implications of the new developments in assisted reproduction.

Yet although the Warnock Report refers to this anxiety at the outset, it is questionable whether that concern is adequately expressed or responded to in the main body of the Report. Much of that anxiety concerns the fate of those created by the artificial techniques: firstly embryos, and secondly children who are destined to become adults. It concerns the implications of this highly unusual start to human life for one's treatment and well-being thereafter. And it is an entirely pertinent criticism of the Warnock Committee that in their desire to meet the needs of adults caught in the distress of infertility they were insufficiently attentive to the likely effects that creation through artificial means has on the child itself. Of course conjecture about these effects is bound to be speculative, partly because many of the techniques are still in their infancy, and partly because one which has been around much longer (AID) has been shrouded in secrecy. Yet research has been done on AID families, and while it has unearthed many stories of apparently happy families with no regrets, it has also brought to light some sad tales which should act as warning lights to couples contemplating this or similar practices.[2]

In the paragraphs which follow I suggest certain ways in which children conceived through artificial techniques may be at risk. I stress the words 'may' and 'at risk'; the undesirable effects envisaged will certainly not ensue in every case. Also, many children conceived through natural means are exposed to similar or comparable risks. But it is surely salutary to consider these dangers.

The first factor is one that might be expected to work to the child's advantage, but could quite conceivably act against it. While the conception of many children is planned by their parents, they are not deliberately and consciously brought into being in the way that artificially created children are. In a natural conception a child is the offshoot of an act in which two partners are interested principally in each other. Ironically, the fate of a child who has been so earnestly desired and deliberately fashioned may be that *too much* love and attention are focussed upon him or her. A child which falls short of expectations may then have a heavy burden to bear.

[1] *Warnock Report,* 1.1.

[2] See R. Snowden and G. D. Mitchell, *The Artificial Family: A Consideration of Artificial Insemination by Donor* (Allen & Unwin, 1981).

Secondly, the fact that the child has been *made* rather than *begotten* may lead one to think of it less as a gift than a possession. The child is the product of ingenious scientific manipulation human gametes. Is it then liable to be thought of as an object which one has at one's disposal? This is probably less of a temptation for parents in relating to their artificially created children than for scientists deciding what to do with embryos in the laboratory. Because the scientists have 'made' the embryo, they appear to feel significantly more free to use it to further human knowledge than would be the case with embryos conceived through natural means.

Thirdly, the peculiarity of the artificially created child's origins expose it to the risk of being a person with obscure and insecure *roots.* Of course, the nature of its conception may be hidden from the child, but this brings its own perils in terms of the strain which keeping an intimate secret imposes on the couple concerned, and such deception is itself morally dubious. However, if the fact that a 'social' parent is not the 'natural' parent is revealed, the disclosure *is* likely to prove traumatic to the child. How deep the disturbance will prove to be depends on a whole range of psychological variables. The same sort of considerations also apply to adopted children, and for some the social acceptability of adoption and the apparent comparability of the family situations are sufficient to render objections to AID and other practices invalid. But there is a crucial difference: in the case of adoption the rootless child has already been created, and the act of adoption contains an element of response to the need of a child whose natural parents cannot give it the stable, loving environment which every child ought to have. Adoption involves the wrenching apart of a natural parental bond, but it happens when the prospects for the child are *nevertheless* thought to be better if this takes place. In the case of 'human assisted reproduction' (to use Lady Warnock's phrase), a child with unusual (and possibly, in part at least, anonymous) genetic roots has been created deliberately. In a world where all too many children seem to suffer crises of identity through confusion about their origins, is it entirely responsible to add to their number?

These caveats, speculative as to some extent they are, do not constitute decisive grounds for rejecting the artificial aids to reproduction *en masse.* However, I believe that they are important considerations, which raise major questions about our society and our culture. The Warnock Committee was understandably wary about exploring them but also seriously negligent in failing to do so.

Hidden amidst the psychological issues of parenting, by natural or artificial means, lie more distinctively ethical questions which demand attention. These concern the separation of procreation from the act of sexual intercourse, and the use of a third party to bring about the desired conception. I shall consider these questions in the course of commenting on different techniques reviewed by the Warnock Report. The techniques are sufficiently different to warrant being treated on their individual merits; at the same time there are comments of a general nature which apply across a range of techniques.

[1] The contrast between making and begetting children is well brought out by Oliver O'Donovan in *Begotten or Made?* (OUP, 1984).

3. CHILDREN WITHOUT SEX?

Amongst the various artificial techniques discussed in the Warnock Report, artificial insemination by husband might be described as the simplest and *in vitro* fertilization as the most advanced, from a technological viewpoint. They occupy opposite ends on the complexity spectrum. But AIH and IVF (as I shall call them henceforth) resemble each other in the fact that the child created is produced from the sperm and eggs of the couple desiring the child; no donation from a third party is involved.[1] AIH entails the injection into a woman's vagina or uterus of her husband's semen. It may be used in cases of the husband's low sperm-count, his physical disability or the wife's cervical hostility. IVF involves the fertilization of a wife's egg (extracted from her ovary) by the husband's semen in a glass dish—not a test-tube!—followed by implantation of the embryo into her uterus. Initially it was almost always used in cases of a woman having blocked or damaged fallopian tubes, but there is now an increasing trend to use it as an alternative to AIH in cases of a man having a low sperm-count. AIH is a simple (though not statistically very successful) procedure which could even be attempted by a couple without the assistance of medical personnel. IVF leaves a couple very much dependent on the Drs. Edwards and Steptoes of this world. But with both techniques, the couple can rest content with the knowledge that the child is entirely theirs, genetically speaking; they have simply taken rather roundabout ways to create it.[1]

The moral issue which confronts us here, then, is the separation of the act of procreation from that of sexual intercourse. The semen which has been produced for the purpose of procreation has been ejaculated not in the act of intercourse but through the act of masturbation. Procreation has become a two- (or more-) stage process where normally it is one. Is this acceptable?

Christians of a modern era would surely agree that it is one of the great glories of God's creation that in sexual intercourse relational and procreational possibilities come together, i.e., the same act can both be a supreme expression of marital love and the beginnings of human life. God has joined these two goods together, and for some Christians any attempt to seek either goal (the supreme expression of marital love or the procreation of children) separately is wrong. Thus Roman Catholics who follow their traditional strand of moral theology would object equally to the use of artificial contraceptives to pursue the relational goal alone and the use of AIH to pursue the procreational goal alone.

However, there is a strong counter-argument that while God has joined these two goods together, couples are not morally obliged to seek both of them equally all the time. Indeed, even with perfectly fertile couples, the occurrence of the menstrual cycle and the passage of time will mean that many acts of intercourse contain little or no potential for the creation

[1] This is true of the simplest and most common form of IVF, but there are complicated variants, which are described in ch. 4.

[2] *More* roundabout in the case of IVF, because the child is actually conceived there outside the woman's body.

of a child. God through nature separates love-making and child-begetting to some extent. The use of contraceptives may be seen as an extension or refinement of means of birth control already present in nature. Nevertheless, because God has provided the potential for achieving procreation through intercourse, one may still be justified in saying that those who persistently use contraceptives to frustrate this end are spurning one of life's great goods.[1] That would be to separate the relational and the procreational so completely as to *exclude* the latter. But a powerful case can still be made for the partial separation of the two on occasion.

As we turn from the issue of contraception to the parallel issues of AIH and IVF, we see that the separation of the two goods here need only be partial. If a husband produces his sperm with the aid of pornographic stimuli, one has to conclude that the marital context of procreation has been lost to view. But ejaculation may occur within the context of a loving sexual encounter with his wife, the climax of which takes a form different from intercourse. There is surely nothing morally objectionable about this? We must resist the tendency of our age to reduce the notion of sexual relationship and encounter simply to the act of sexual intercourse. If there is a grounding of the production of gametes within the sexual relationship, then the two goods which, in the case of the physically impaired (not infertile) couple have *not* been perfectly joined together, are at least being held in conjunction. With regard to provision of suitable time and place for such couples medical services ought to bear such considerations in view. This is another delicate psychological and moral area on which the Warnock Report is silent.

In principle, then, and subject to the qualifications of the last paragraph, AIH and IVF are acceptable. But that acceptance is qualified by additional considerations relating to the two practices.

The Warnock Report itself records grave misgivings about AIH in one type of situation. This is where a man who knows he is destined soon to die donates his semen and his wife seeks insemination after his death.[1] Here a deliberate decision is being made to create a child who from the very start will only have one parent. While some single parents cope marvellously well when forced into that role by circumstances like divorce or bereavement, children *are* best served by having two parents, a mother and a father. Deliberately to create an AIH child without a father is a clear case of irresponsible procreation—because the circumstances into which it will be born are known in advance to be far from ideal.

Misgivings about IVF are more substantial because they relate to the way in which it is practised normally, not exceptionally. IVF has only reached its present sophisticated stage of development because of the many embryos which were used as 'guinea-pigs' at an earlier stage. Conception takes place outside the womb: this raises moral questions about what to do with embryos observed to be defective or with surplus

[1] This is a general, not a universal judgment. The circumstances of some couples (e.g. carrying a hereditary condition, or marrying in one's late 30s) are such that they might constitute an exception.

[2] A widely publicized example of this happened in France.

embryos produced because the woman's ovaries have been stimulated artificially. More will be said about the status of the embryo and its implications for IVF in chapter 5.

If the chapter-title of 'Children Without Sex?' is actually a little unfair with regard to sexually active couples who resort to AIH and IVF, it is more appropriate in relation to the demand made by some homosexual and lesbian couples to have access to the artificial techniques. They do have a sexual relationship but not one in which intercourse in the normal sense of the word takes place, nor one in which there is any hope of procreating from within the relationship. If the use of artificial techniques were to be allowed in this context, the disruption of the connection between sexual intercourse and procreation could not be more complete. Children would be being provided on order for individuals who had set themselves against the possibility of conceiving children by natural means. The Warnock Report was right to disallow this possibility.[1]

[1] See *Warnock Report,* 2.11.

4. A MULTIPLICATION OF PARENTS

When a child is conceived, born and reared, in the usual way, husband and wife provide the sperm and the egg respectively; the wife carries and bears the child; and the husband and wife bring the child up. Just the two individuals are involved in playing these different crucial roles in parenting. Artificial techniques have now been developed to a stage where no less than five different individuals may take part, and, depending on who plays which part, a total of 11 different combinations of technique and 'parent' are possible. They are as follows:

(i) Artificial Insemination by Donor (AID)
This is the most common. A donor provides the sperm, the wife is inseminated and bears the child, the wife and her husband act as social parents. It is used in cases of the husband's sterility or significantly low sperm-count, and for avoidance of hereditary diseases where these are carried by the male. Three individuals involved.

(ii) Surrogate Motherhood without IVF
Another woman is inseminated with the sperm of the husband, and carries the child until birth on the understanding that she will then give it up to the husband and wife who will be its social parents. It may be used when the wife is both infertile and incapable of carrying the child. There individuals involved.

(iii) Egg Donation by Lavage
Another woman is inseminated with the sperm of the husband. Three or four days after fertilization her uterus is washed out (*lavage*), and the embryo is transferred to the uterus of the wife, who then carries it. As in every case, the husband and wife will be the social parents. It may be used when the wife is infertile. Three individuals involved.

(iv) Embryo Donation by Lavage
An egg donor is inseminated with sperm from another donor. Her uterus is then washed out and the embryo transferred to the wife. It may be used in rare cases where both husband and wife are infertile. Four individuals involved.

(v) Sperm Donation by IVF
An egg from the wife is fertilized by a sperm donor *in vitro,* and the resulting embryo is implanted in the wife. This might be used in cases of the husband's infertility if AID has not worked. Three individuals involved.

(iv) Egg Donation by IVF
A female donor provides the egg which is fertilized *in vitro* by the husband's sperm. The embryo is inplanted in the wife. Three individuals involved.

(vii) Embryo Donation by IVF
A donated egg is fertilized *in vitro* with donated sperm (or the embryo may be a 'spare' one from another couple on an IVF programme). The embryo is implanted in the wife. As with (iv), this may be used where both husband and wife are infertile. Four individuals involved.

(viii) Surrogate Motherhood by IVF
A wife's egg is fertilized *in vitro* with the husband's sperm. The embryo is then transferred to the uterus of another woman, who carries it until birth for the couple. This might be used where the wife is unable to sustain a pregnancy, and in preference to (ii) if IVF proved more successful than artificial insemination in leading to fertilization. Three individuals involved.

(ix) Surrogate Motherhood by Sperm Donation and IVF
A wife's egg is fertilized *in vitro* with a donor's sperm. The embryo is transferred to another woman, who carries it for the couple. This might be used where the husband is infertile and the wife unable to sustain a pregnancy. Four individuals involved.

(x) Surrogate Motherhood by Egg Donation and IVF
A donated egg is fertilized *in vitro* with the husband's sperm. The embryo is then carried by a woman other than the donor. This might be used where the wife is infertile and incapable of carrying a child. Four individuals (including three women!) involved.

(xi) Surrogate Motherhood by Sperm Donation, Egg Donation and IVF
This is the same as (x) with the added complication that the husband is infertile, necessitating a sperm donor. Five individuals involved.

Clearly we are confronted by a staggering plethora of possibilities! In fact, some of these combinations are extremely unlikely, have not to my knowledge occurred in this country, and are not considered explicitly by the Warnock Report, notably examples (ix)-(xi). The two types of surrogate motherhood most likely to occur are (ii) and (viii).

The Warnock Committee would also like to restrict the range of possibilities by banning, for the time being at least, the use of 'lavage'. This is because of the risk of pregnancy in the donor, since the embryo may not be washed out, or of the introduction of infection to her uterus. If the technique became safer, it seems they would be willing to allow it.[1]

With regard to the remaining, already well established practices, different techniques may or may not be deemed acceptable, depending on one's answer to the following questions:

> If a technique involves IVF, is it morally flawed by the association of that programme with experiments on embryos?[2]
> If a technique involves surrogate motherhood, does that represent the intrusion of a third party more serious than that involved in the donation of sperm and egg?
> If a technique involves both types of donation, does that make it better or worse than involving simply sperm or egg?
> Finally, is the principle of any third party intervention at all ethically acceptable?

[1] *Warnock Report,* 7.5.
[2] I discuss this in ch. 5.

Techniques involving surrogacy are notable for comprising the one category of artificial techniques which the Warnock Committee, excepting a minority of two, decided to oppose.[1] While recognizing that the bearing of a child for another couple may be an act of genuine generosity, and that surrogate mothers generally enter into the transaction thoughtfully and with every intention of returning the child to the couple concerned, the Report brings forward powerful counter-arguments to allowing such a practice. Most surrogacy agreements involve a commercial element. On the one hand the surrogate mother (and of course a commercial agency) may exploit the couple: '. . . it is inconsistent with human dignity that a woman should use her uterus for financial profit and treat it as an incubator for someone else's child.[2] On the other hand the couple may exploit the woman: pregnancy involves risks, and that 'people should treat others as a means to their own ends, however desirable the consequences, must always be liable to moral objection.'[3] Furthermore, the intrusion of a third party into the marital relationship is much greater than with AID, egg donation or embryo donation, because the surrogate mother actually carries the baby for nine months and then bears it. During that period one can expect a considerable degree of bonding between child-bearer and child to take place, so that it may well be a considerable wrench for the woman to give up the child. Whatever the previous agreement they have entered into, women should not be made subject to mental and emotional anguish of this sort.

My own view is that this personal and intimate character of the bonding process constitutes the most weighty reason for prohibiting surrogacy. The commercial consideration cannot *per se* be decisive because provision could be made for a non-commercial surrogacy service (as Drs. Greengross and Davies in their minority report suggested). It is the ruling out of order of that most basic of a mother's desires—to keep the child she has just born—which is fundamentally objectionable. Surrogacy is playing with fire.

The technique of embryo donation has also come in for criticism from some quarters. The Warnock Committee, while allowing it, deemed embryo donation 'probably the least satisfactory form of donation'[4] (for reasons undisclosed). The Church of England BSR Working Party which responded to the Warnock Report decided by a small majority that it exceeded the permitted bounds within which man through technology may seek to alter the course of nature; they thought that the implantation in a woman of an embryo with no genetic relationship to either her or her husband 'entails treating that child too much as a product'.[5] I have discovered other examples of embryo donation being deemed to be inhuman, impersonal and clinically anonymous by those who carefully exclude such adjectives from description of sperm or egg donation.

[1] See *Warnock Report,* ch. 8 and Expression of Dissent A.
[2] *Op. cit.,* 8.10.
[3] *Op. cit.,* 8.17.
[4] *Op. cit.,* 7.4.
[5] *Personal Origins* (CIO, 1985) p.46.

Personally, I find such a distinction hard to accept. The minority on the BSR Working Party judged that

> 'the distinction between implanting an embryo with a donated ovum, one with donated semen, and one where both ovum and semen are donated, seems one of degree. Once the principle of donation is granted, some would see little reason to insist that at least 50 per cent of the embryo's genes should be those of one social parent.'[1]

I would add that embryo donation can be seen as having an advantage over AID and egg donation. The fact that husband and wife stand in an equivalent, non-existent genetic relationship to the child means that emotional bonds with the child are likely to be of similar strength. The situation thus has similarities with that of adoption, so that some would even describe it as *pre-natal* adoption. Nevertheless, a crucial dissimilarity with adopting couples remains, in that the latter involves responding to the needs of a child who lacks a proper home, whereas embryo donation entails the deliberate creation of a child with the most anonymous of genetic origins.

Quite apart from the fact that it is rare for both husband and wife to be infertile, and consequently there is little demand for embryo donation, the reason why AID and its female equivalent have found greater favour is the existence here of a genetic link on one side of the parent-child relationship. Where couples who have resorted to AID have also had a chance of adopting, influential considerations have been the desire to create a child which would inherit traits from the wife, the wish to be sure of 50% of 'what they are getting'[2], and the fact that the wife is able to savour the precious experiences of pregnancy and childbirth. These concerns may well weigh as strongly with the husband as the wife. Doctors who have participated in AID procedures thus far appear to be scrupulous about ensuring that husband and wife are united in their desire for a child by this method. It is unfair to describe AID as adultery—as some objectors to the practice have done—because the elements of sexual union with another partner and deliberate unfaithfulness to one's own partner (the essential features of adultery) are clearly absent from AID.

Nevertheless, however much the couple are agreed at the time and however much they think that the birth of a child will benefit their marriage, there is something alien to the spirit and nature of marriage in the concept of AID or egg donation. It is wrong to think of marriage as a purely private relationship which involves no giving to, or receiving from, the wider community; successful marriages are ones where couples are open to help from other people. Yet marriage—by which I mean a Christian view of marriage which still has some reverberations in our increasingly secular culture—is a covenant relationship between husband and wife exclusive of all others in certain key areas of life. The procreation of children stands with sexual intercourse as a personal and intimate activity at the very heart of married life, where it is signally inappropriate to assign a crucial role to an outsider. The logic of the marriage vows ('for

[1] *Op. cit.,* Expression of Dissent B, para. 3.
[2] A phrase used by a husband quoted in *The Artificial Family,* p.34.

better, for *worse,* in *sickness* and in health') appears to imply that the partner who is strong in fertility terms should show solidarity with the partner who is weak where such an important area of marriage is concerned. If it does not, then there is need for serious re-examination of what the promises of faithfulness in marriage do exclude.

When appeal is made to the use of third parties to circumvent infertility in the patriarchal sagas, the social contexts of these stories needs to be borne in mind. Slave-girls were regarded virtually as property; Hagar and Bilhah were seen as assistants to their mistress, and that included the child-creating area if need be. The institution of slavery both makes sense of the patriarchal practice and evokes repugnance, because we feel that slavery is something we have left behind. Abraham and Jacob scarcely provide very precise parallels for the artificial techniques being considered in today's society.

Although research into AID families reveals many couples who harbour no regrets, and where the marriage has remained stable, where problems have occurred they have often been related to the *loss of solidarity* which admission of the AID technique into marriage represents. Sometimes the husband comes to resent the fact that the child is not as much 'his' as his wife's. If marital breakdown occurs for other reasons, the fact that the child was created by AID may still be used by one partner to hurt the other. In one case cited by Snowden and Mitchell a husband resented his wife's desire to have several children by AID.[1]

A further objection to techniques involving third party intervention concerns the part played by the donor. As with surrogacy, the aspect of donors being paid has been called into question. The Warnock Committee showed unease with this, recommending a gradual move towards a system where semen and egg donors would only be given their expenses.[2] It should probably have grasped the nettle and recommended an *immediate* move; it seems that the current difficulty in getting suitable donors deterred them. But if semen donation (the usual type) was devoid of financial reward, it would still be morally questionable, because here the traditional objections to masturbation assume real force. Semen is produced through a process quite divorced from the loving sexual relationship which is its context in the case of AIH.

All in all, the objections to AID and egg donation are at least as substantial as in the case of embryo donation, if not more so—because of the imbalance in relation with the child between husband and wife. Some Christian bodies consider these objections so decisive that they demand that these practices be banned forthwith.[3] But it is at this point that I feel conscious of a gap between what is morally right and what is legally permissible. If the major objections to AID rest on a high, covenantal view of marriage, as they do, we have to be about the fact that many couples in today's society are operating in a looser, less demanding, framework. Their emotional commitment to each other and their desire for a child

[1] *Op. cit.,* p.50.
[2] *Warnock Report,* 3.27.
[3] E.g. CARE Trust and the Catholic Bishops' Joint Committee on Bio-Ethical Issues.

enable them (temporarily, at least) to set aside the restrictions normally implicit in the concept of faithfulness. Because infertility does cause such heartache to many couples, because the large-scale practice of abortion already has drastically reduced the flow of children available for adoption, and because AID at any rate is already a well established technique, it may be appropriate to make provision for gamete donation in this country. Much depends on how wide one thinks the gap between moral ideal enactment should be permitted to be. If one thinks that the moral health of a society is best protected by closing the gap, the moral questionability of techniques involving third party intervention will be sufficient argument for banning them. But if, as I do, one thinks that closing this gap will have the effect of forcing such techniques below the surface of society, where they will be practised in a less principled way, one may be prepared to allow their practice while retaining one's moral reservations.

If one accepts that AID, egg donation and embryo donation should be regularized by law, then many of the Warnock Report's recommendations seem to be along the right lines.[1] It tries to sort out the legal vacuum surrounding AID. The report recommends that the AID child should be treated as the legitimate child of the mother and her husband where they have both consented to treatment, that the law should be changed so that the donor will have no parental rights or duties in relation to the child, and that the husband should be registered as the father. This last recommendation has been criticized as promulgating a legal fiction; in anticipation of this, the Warnock Committee suggested the possibility of adding the words 'by donation' to the birth certificate, but they would have been wiser to exclude all legal deception by insisting on this. Snowden and Mitchell's study brings out clearly the problems which AID couples inflict on themselves (and, potentially, the AID child) by trying to keep the nature of the child's conception a secret.[2] If the child does find out, the fact that the couple have not volunteered the information adds to the trauma. The Warnock Report encourages a lifting of the veil of secrecy over third party practices and indeed recommends that at the age of 18 the child should have access to basic information about the donor's ethnic origin and health. It also stipulates that the number of children produced by any one donor should be limited to 10, in order to reduce the risk of his or her transmitting (unknowingly) an inheritable disease or the remote possibility of unwitting incest between children from the same donor.

A more controversial recommendation of the Warnock Report is that the couple to whom these artificial techniques are available need not necessarily be husband and wife (as, thus far, I have assumed them to be). Their working definition of a couple is 'a heterosexual couple living together in a stable relationship, whether married or not.'[3] This has been strongly attacked from a variety of quarters: compare the late Raymond Johnston on behalf of CARE Trust ('the Warnock Report ignores the God-given pattern of man-woman relationship in marriage as the only right

[1] See *Warnock Report,* 4.17-4.28.

[2] See *The Artificial Family,* chs. 4 and 5.

[3] *Warnock Report,* 2.6.

place for the procreation and care of children'[1]); the Catholic Bishops' Joint Committee on Bio-Ethical Issues ('there is no other relationship which can, for practical purposes, be identified as an appropriate substitute for the environment which a good marriage certainly does provide for the child'[2]); and the Chief Rabbi of Great Britain (not limiting access to treatment for infertility to legally married couples 'would constitute an intolerable affront to the most precious element of the Judeao-Christian heritage, and would cause incalculable harm to children deliberately conceived under such circumstances.'[3]).

Whether one finds these arguments conclusive again depends in part on what one judges to be an appropriate relationship between morality and the law. One can still hold fast to marriage as the right setting for full sexual relations while recognizing that some cohabiting couples do demonstrate a level of emotional stability and long-term commitment to each other which bear comparison with a 'good' marriage. Couples are unlikely to resort to requesting artificial techniques until they have been together several years; long-term commitment is therefore likely to characterize such relationships, whether marital or not, and of course many couples who begin by cohabiting do marry within a few years. I suspect that the number of couples requesting artificial techniques who are not married is small, and that because it is no longer possible to measure depth of commitment by the presence or absence of a marriage certificate it would be unfair to exclude them automatically.

[1] This quotation is taken from a piece of CARE campaign literature behind which I detect Raymond's influence.

[2] *Response to the Warnock Report* (Catholic Media Office, 1984), pp.10-11.

[3] Immanuel Jakobovits, 'Warnock: ethics undermined' in *The Times,* 15 December 1984.

5. EMBRYOS—HUMAN BEINGS OR GUINEA PIGS?

Of all the artificial techniques discussed in the Warnock Report, *in vitro* fertilization is the one that has attracted most public attention. 'Test-tube' babies have been acclaimed as a marvel of scientific ingenuity; media coverage has been overwhelmingly favourable towards the practice. As we have seen, IVF usually avoids the moral complication of using gametes from a third party. Surely it is one technique about which we can be whole-heartedly enthusiastic? But the fact is that the processes involved in IVF make it the most questionable of all these techniques.

Admittedly, most of the moral scruples focus around a judgment which is a matter of some controversy, the status of the human embryo. In coming out against surrogacy, the Warnock Report made much of the traditional moral argument that human beings should not be treated as a means to other people's ends, however great the benefit to the latter might be. But if the early embryo is a human being—or even, as I shall argue, if its status is nearly akin to that—one is obliged to acknowledge that IVF has involved and still involves the using of human beings as a means to other people's ends on a vast scale. Between 1969 and 1978 Dr. Robert Edwards and Mr. Patrick Steptoe developed and then destroyed hundreds of human embryos in their attempt to perfect a technique to which they felt confident about subjecting a would-be mother. These embryos were effectively 'guinea-pigs'. In the years since 1978 embryos have continued to be used experimentally in order to refine the technique and improve its success-rate. One way of increasing the likelihood of success is to give the woman fertility drugs. A typical situation which ensues is one in which six eggs are produced, and fertilized with the husband's sperm. All may develop into embryos. Two might be implanted in the wife; two might be 'frozen' for possible use at a future date; two (probably ones which do not appear to be developing normally) might be used for observation and research. These are the so-called *spare embryos.*

The research which is practised and envisaged is of various types. First, there are experiments which are therapeutic in the sense that they are designed to bring benefit to other people, but are lethal as far as the embryo itself is concerned. Thus a gene from a healthy embryo might be transplanted into an embryo which had been discovered through screening to be genetically defective, or cells from an embryo might be grafted into patients with bone marrow or diabetic disorders. Secondly, there are experiments designed to identify whether parents known to have a significant statistical risk of producing children with genetic defects have in fact done so: an early embryo can be split ('twinned'), one twin then tested for defects, and, if it 'passes', the other twin then replaced in the mother. If it fails, both parts of the embryc are destroyed. Similarly, where a genetic disease is linked to the sex of a child, an embryo whose sex has been determined could be replaced or destroyed accordingly. Thirdly, some scientists would like to test drugs on embryos rather than animals. Fourthly, there is the hope that through doing tests more will be discovered about why so many early embryos miscarry naturally, with the long-term hope of reducing the miscarriage rate significantly, and thereby also reducing the number of couples who are naturally childless.

All these aims sound very worthy, and yet the chilling fact is that experimentation on an embryo almost always entails inflicting lethal harm on it. Others may (either in the short- or, more likely, very long-term) benefit, but the embryo subject to research will not. Only in a very limited number of cases do experiments not inflict any harm on the embryo and hence there is a possibility of it being implanted in its mother.

I do not have space here to do justice to all aspects of the debate surrounding the status of the embryo. The Warnock Report fails dismally to enter properly into this debate at all:

> 'Although the questions of when life or personhood begin to appear to be questions of fact susceptible of straighforward answers, we hold that the answers to such questions in fact are complex amalgams of factual and moral judgments. Instead of trying to answer these questions directly we have therefore gone straight to the question of *how it is right to treat the human embryo.'*[1]

This is lamentable on two counts. First, the Warnock Committee dodged the key question: how could they decide the right way to treat the human embryo when they were undecided what its status is? Secondly, 'life or personhood' and 'factual and moral' are two ill-chosen couplets. The question of when life begins is susceptible of a straightforward factual answer. What is present from the moment of fertilization is unquestionably alive. It is an organism in the process of growth and development. And it is alive in a significantly different sense from the pre-fertilization sperm and egg because (unlike either of those separately) it has the potential to develop into a creature whom we would all describe as a human person. Whether personhood should already be ascribed to the early embryo is a more open question, but it is not so much a moral judgment as an evaluative one.

The word 'personhood' itself eludes precise or generally agreed definition. But what is fundamentally at stake is whether the embryo commands a status and deserves a respect comparable to that given to human persons outside the womb. In short, is status linked to attainment of a particular stage in the developmental process? Developmental progress is not linked to sanctity of life outside the womb: to kill a two-hour-old baby is as much murder as to kill a sportsman at the height of his powers or an old-age pensioner. All would be equally protected under the Declaration of Helsinki from research which might do them lethal harm. So from the evaluative judgment about whether early embryos possess similar status follow moral judgments about whether research on them is permissible.

As the debate since the publication of the Warnock Report has made clear, Christians, especially in the Church of England, are seriously divided over whether the early embryo is a person or not. It is a question to which neither the Bible nor Christian tradition give a transparently unambiguous answer. Certainly there are biblical passages which suggest a high view of life in the womb, and in which the writers' conviction that it was he, the same person, who was the object of God's prenatal creative activity and care shines through clearly.[2] But these

[1] *Warnock Report*, 11.0.

[2] See e.g. Psalm 139.13-16, Job 10.8-12, Jer. 1.5.

passages do not definitely have the embryo in its earliest stages in view[1]; and there is one passage which, if translated and interpreted in a certain way, appears to rank post-natal life more highly than pre-natal life.[2] Again, though Christian tradition has been united, until very recent times, in regarding the deliberate taking of fetal life with horror, it has divided over the precise status of the fetus at different stages in development. One strand of opinion has insisted on the full personal status of the embryo from the time of conception. This strand is reflected in the BSR report minority view, which took as its point of reference the *continuity of the individual subject,* however hidden that 'someone' may be in the earliest stages.[3] The other strand of opinion ha argued that the fetus is not animated by a soul until some way into pregnancy—40 days in the case of a male. This viewpoint does not find precise expression in the BSR report majority view, since the concept of 'soul' as a substantive entity is increasingly hard to justify, but they identify a similar key point of discontinuity in the emergence of a *subject of consciousness.* The majority group linked this to a particular stage in brain development, 'the emergence of a functioning nerve-net'[4] which they date, interestingly enough, at around 40 days. Their judgment on the status of the embryo is therefore similar in essential respects to that of the majority on the Warnock Committee. The latter was anxious not to permit research on embryos whose central nervous system was beginning to develop (about 23 days) and might thus experience pain; subtracting a few days to be on the safe side, they arrived at 15 days, a point which coincides with the development of the primitive streak.[5] Before then, the majority groups on both Warnock Committee and BSR Working Party are prepared to allow research where worthy aims can only be realized through it.

Personally, I believe that the present fashionable obsession with brain development is precisely that—a fashionable obsession. Which particular stage in brain development one considers to be crucial differs widely from one judge to another. The BSR Working Party was confident that function activity starts around 40 days; the Warnock Committee, more modestly and more accurately, said that the timing is unknown. Measurement of embryonic brain activity by EEG reveals no consistent pattern. Since it is the *potential* (i.e., the potential to think, articulate, decide) of the brain which obviously attracts the advocates of this viewpoint, it is illogical that they choose neither to wait for the moment when the child actually shows evidence of doing such things—in which case they might be waiting till the time when he or she goes to playgroup!—nor to respect the potential which is contained within the embryo from the outset. In fact the whole preoccupation with man's rationality is symptomatic of our secular, post-Enlightenment age, and it is disappointing to find so many Christians jumping on this particular bandwagon. God's love for man and the glory of God as reflected—'imaged'—in man do not depend fundamentally on the fact that man has (analogous to God, presumably) a highly complex brain.

[1] Not that there is any reason for thinking the biblical writers would exclude it!

[2] Ex. 21.22-25. But the sense is altered radically by whether a miscarriage is referred to (see RSV translation) or a premature birth (see NIV).

[3] For expression of the two views, see *Personal Origins,* ch. 3.

[4] *Op. cit.,* p.29.

[5] See *Warnock Report,* 11.19-11.22.

I am driven to the conclusion that to choose any point other than fertilization for ascribing human status to the embryo is highly arbitrary. There are of course arguments regularly lodged against taking this step. For instance, a great many fertilized eggs miscarry at an early age, sometimes even before a woman knows that she is pregnant. Can these really be persons who have perished? The answer 'yes' is not as silly as at first it may sound. The history of the world is full of infants who have perished early, at birth or soon after, and their personal status goes unquestioned; the phenomenon of natural miscarriage simply shows a similar sort of occurrence happening even earlier. The fact that cell division to produce twinning may occur up to 14 days after fertilization is used as an argument against stress on the embryo's genetic uniqueness from the point of fusion. Yet a cell destined to 'twin' retains its genetic *particularity;* that particularity may well determine the fact that it will split; and perhaps the best way to describe it at its earliest stage is two persons under the *appearance* of being one. Another argument is that parents do not usually *feel* a great loss when a miscarriage happens very early; the embryo or fetus is felt to be more of a person the longer it survives. This is true, yet we need to be extremely careful what conclusions we draw from people's feelings. The mother of an eight-week-old fetus who wants an abortion is likely to feel it is less of a person than the mother of an eight-week-old fetus who wants a baby. But if the first girl was to see her fetus on scan, her feelings might well change. Yet the extent of the fetus' development would be the same in all three cases. We ought to put more trust in the objective scientific data than our own limited powers of imagination in trying to determine whether the embryo is a person or not.

Granted that the imagination does baulk at the data, it is understandable that some people are willing to describe the early embryo only in terms of a potential person. What conclusions follow from there is unpredictable. Type A includes and stresses the word *only* potential, and assumes that experiments on embryos are therefore permissible. Type B insists that we must still treat the embryo with great reverence and respect, but still finds the resource of courage (or cowardice?) to permit experiments under 'strict ethical criteria'. The majority on the BSR Working Party comprised Type B. Type C takes the notion of potential seriously, and refuses to allow embryo research. The minority group on the Warnock Committee who dissented from research did so on the grounds that

> 'the embryo has a special status because of its potential for development to a stage at which everyone would accord it the status of a human person. It is in our view wrong to create something with the potential for becoming a human person and then deliberately to destroy it.'[1]

Just as children with the potential for an active electoral or political life suffer injustice if, through a change in political system, they never get the chance to exercise it, so an embryo can suffer the most serious form of injustice, undeserved death, even if it never consciously experiences dying.

Opposition to the practice of embryo research need not be limited, then, to those who are convinced that the early embryo is *already* a person. It

[1] *Op. cit.,* Expression of Dissent B, para. 3.

can and does also take in those who think the embryo *may* be a person (since it is irresponsible to risk killing someone) and some of those who regard it as a potential person. However, the research practitioners are going to prove very difficult to stop. To be fair, some of them do appear to share some of the moral hesitations evident in e.g., the BSR Working Party. Thus Edwards and Steptoe would prefer to restrict experiments to embryos which are the by-products of their IVF technique; they stress that these embryos are 'no-hopers',[1] ones with no hope of survival in a human womb, and since they are already doomed, what does it matter if we hasten their end a little and in the process accumulate some useful knowledge? But embryo research cannot be justified so easily. First, if the embryo is doomed to perish soon, ought it not to be allowed a peaceful death? The fact that certain elderly patients are racked by terminal cancer is no excuse for performing lethal experiments on them. Secondly, if the researchers stumbled across a 'spare' embryo which was not defective in any way, but would—if implanted in a suitable environment—have a fair chance of development, would they really be inhibited about doing research on it? One suspects not. Indeed, the Warnock Committee by the smallest of majorities approved the creation of embryos specifically for research purposes. These would include many healthy embryos, and for certain types of research, that is precisely the sort of embryo which is required. Restriction of research to Steptoe's 'no-hopers' would not suit many scientists; nor is it feasible that a distinction between embryos which, given a uterine environment, *do* have a chance of survival (on which experiments should not be done) and embryos which do *not* (on which they may) could be maintained either in practice or at law. It is also relevant to point out that some scientists are irked by the possibility of the 14-day limit recommended by Warnock; they want freedom to perform experiments for at least twice that length.

The drift of my argument against IVF will now be painfully clear. I say 'painfully' because I would genuinely prefer not to be driven to an adverse judgment on a technique which has brought joy and promises hope for certain types of infertile couples. Some will say: if IVF was practised in a way which involved no lethal experiments, i.e., if the women were not superovulated, so that there were no spare embryos, or if any research done was strictly therapeutic (i.e., of benefit to the embryo on whom it was being done), surely IVF would be acceptable? I would like to clutch at this straw, but honesty forbids it. IVF practised in this self-denying way would have its already low success rate cut to a point where it became prohibitively expensive. Although the technique may soon be reaching its upper limit of improvement, some practitioners will continue to want embryos which they do not intend to implant to pave the way for those they do so intend. And if the solitary egg which has been fertilized appears malformed, is one morally bound to implant it? Probably not; and yet to be saddled in a laboratory with an embryo which one can responsibly neither help to live nor help to die is an invidious (and itself irresponsible) position in which to put oneself. There are moral dilemmas right at the heart of the IVF process, not just the process in the way that it has developed.

[1] This is a phrase used by Patrick Steptoe in a debate in which I participated at the Cambridge Union.

6. THE WEAKNESS OF WARNOCK

When confronted by the Warnock issues, people often react in one of two opposite ways. The first is to throw up one's hands in horror at the technological manipulation of human beginnings and demand that those who sadly are childless live within creaturely limits. The second is to rejoice at man's capacity to transcend those limits and submit to the fascinating lure that techniques like AID and IVF undoubtedly hold. In other words, one often encounters an 'all or nothing' response. Either they are all wrong, or they are all acceptable.

Like the Warnock Committee, I have seen fit to steer a middle path, to distinguish between techniques which are morally or socially acceptable and those which are not. To make such distinctions may appear very unfair to those whose disability leaves them with recourse only to a technique which is deemed unacceptable. Yet a readiness to give assent to any artificial technique, however grotesque it might be and whatever the cost, is clearly unsupportable, unless one believes that the relief of childlessness is a moral priority which supplants all others. If that is so, then we are saying more than that couples *want* children and *need* children; we are saying that they have an absolute *right* to children.

However, we cannot responsibly consider the problems of childlessness in isolation from other moral considerations and social constraints. The sacrifice of countless embryos at the altar of IVF cannot simply be ignored. A major expansion of infertility services such as Warnock envisages raises serious question about medical priorities. I am not saying that the infertile should not be on the priorities list; but in an age of financial cut-backs, it is not clear that they should be substantially further up the list.

The Warnock Report and I part company in where we set our limits at various points. One would like to be clearer about why *it* sets its limits where it does. A major criticism of the Committee is that having summed up the pros and cons of a particular argument, they fail to explain satisfactorily why they decided on their point of view. Too often it seems to be because they deemed it 'the more generally held position'; sometimes it is a case of a bald 'we recommend' or an inadequately explained 'we have reached the conclusion'.[1] But inasmuch as one can surmise about the philosophy behind the Report, two characteristics emerge. One is the utilitarian drift. Despite the principled stand that it takes over surrogacy, the lure of future benefits and the minimization of pain swayed the majority over embryo research. The second is its seduction by the technological spirit of the age and unwillingness to accept limits beyond which man should never go. As I have noted, its discussion of the problems faced by childless couples is deficient in attention to non-technological considerations. The Report is surprisingly ambivalent about the possibity of parents selecting the sex of children for purely social reasons in the future.[2] It appreciates public anxiety about the possibility of ectogenesis or selective breeding and anticipates that the

[1] For examples of these phrases see *Warnock Report, paras. 11.15, 12.9 and 5.10.*
[2] *Op. cit.,* paras. 9.11-9.12.

licensing body it proposes will ban them; yet readily assumes that the guidance given by the body will be 'reviewed from time to time to take account of both changes in scientific knowledge and changes in public attitudes'.[1] While the Warnock Committee could not ignore public attitudes in making legal recommendations, and while the harshest critics of the Report are open to the charge of doing precisely that, the Report does give the impression of being too much at the beck and call of public attitudes. It could have been expected to give more of a moral lead. Sadly, the present Government shows no indication of filling the gap and doing so.

[1] *Op. cit.,* para. 12.16.